Herbal Skin Solutions

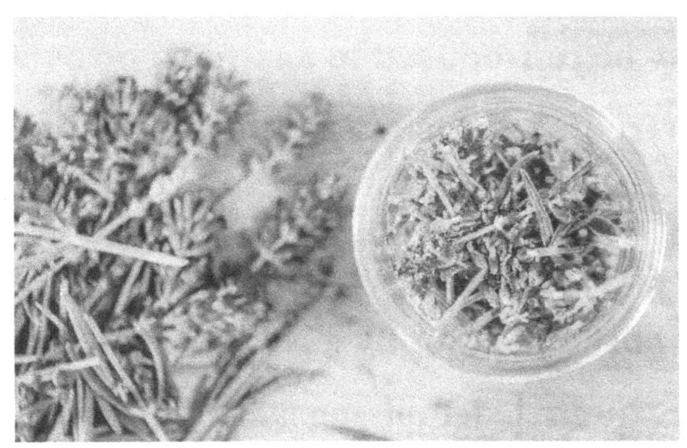

The Ultimate Guide to Natural Remedies for Acne, Eczema, ageing skin and Psoriasis

Charles K. Borrego

Copyright© 2023 by Charles K. Borrego

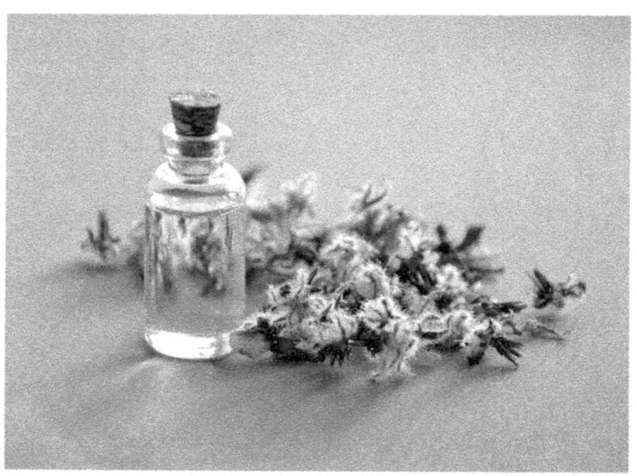

Table of contents

Introduction

Chapter 1: The Benefits of herbal remedies for Skin Conditions

Chapter 2: Treating Acne with Herbal Remedies

    A 7-day Herbal Recipes Plan

Chapter 3: Treating Eczema with Herbal Remedies

    A 7-day Herbal Recipes Plan

Chapter 4: Treating Ageing Skin with Herbal Remedies

    A 7-day Herbal Recipes Plan

Chapter 5: Treating Psoriasis with herbal remedies

    A 7-day Herbal Recipes Plan

Chapter 6: Treating Burns and Sunburns with Herbal Remedies

    Types of Burns and Sunburns

    Herbal Remedies for Burns and Sunburns

    A 7-day Herbal Recipes Plan

Chapter 7: Treating Hyperpigmentation with herbal remedies

    A 7-day Herbal Recipes Plan

Conclusion

Introduction

Herbal remedies have become part of the essential toolkit for treating various skin conditions due to their natural ingredients and efficacy. For thousands of years, various cultures have relied on herbal remedies to treat a variety of ailments and skin conditions. These remedies are not limited to any particular culture or age group, but offer a wide range of treatments for people of all ages and backgrounds. Herbal remedies for skin conditions have the potential to relieve dryness, reduce inflammation, balance oil production, fight bacteria, and keep the skin looking healthy and youthful. They are widely available, safe, and can be used effectively in the treatment of a wide range of common and uncommon skin conditions.

Herbal remedies offer a natural option for treating, healing, and calming the skin without the use of harsh chemicals and synthetic ingredients. Many herbs have natural anti-inflammatory, antifungal, antibacterial, and antioxidant properties, making them beneficial for the overall health of the skin. Additionally, herbal extracts are often more easily absorbed by the body than topical ointments, providing an added layer of protection to the skin cells.

By properly obtaining and utilising herbal remedies for skin conditions, individuals can obtain long-term relief from their symptoms without the need for expensive and potentially harmful drugs. With the correct application and dosage of herbal treatments, individuals can experience improved skin health, comfort, and accelerated healing of their skin condition. Herbal remedies provide an affordable, accessible, and natural approach to skin care, and can be used with other traditional treatments to maintain and improve long-term skin health.

Chapter 1: The Benefits of herbal remedies for Skin Conditions

Herbal remedies are becoming increasingly popular as a natural alternative to conventional medicines for various skin conditions. Herbal medicines are derived from plants and can be used to treat a wide variety of ailments, including skin disorders. Herbal remedies offer many potential benefits, including being easy to use and generally safe, with few side effects.

Herbal remedies have been used for centuries to treat skin issues. They can work in many ways, depending on the plant and its properties. Some herbs can reduce redness, itching, and inflammation while others can boost immunity and fight off bacteria or fungi. Herbal remedies can also promote faster healing and help prevent reoccurrence of the condition.

One of the biggest benefits of herbal remedies is that they're easy to find and use. There are many herbal medicine brands that are available both online and in stores that can provide a wide variety of herbs for different skin conditions. Many people also grow their own herbs, which makes it easy and economical to get the exact herbs they need.

Another benefit to using herbal remedies for skin conditions is that they're generally safe. Herbal remedies are usually used as topical applications and, if used correctly, can cause few, if any, side effects. When using herbal remedies, it's important to be aware of potential interactions with medications, as some herbal medicines can have interactions with other drugs.

Herbal treatments can also be less expensive than conventional medicines, making them an attractive option for those on a tight budget. Additionally, some herbs are known to have many health benefits beyond treating skin conditions, such as helping to reduce stress, improve sleep, improve digestion, and more.

Overall, herbal remedies can be an excellent choice for people dealing with skin issues that want to use a more natural approach. Herbal remedies are easy to use, generally safe, and can provide significant relief and healing for many different skin conditions.

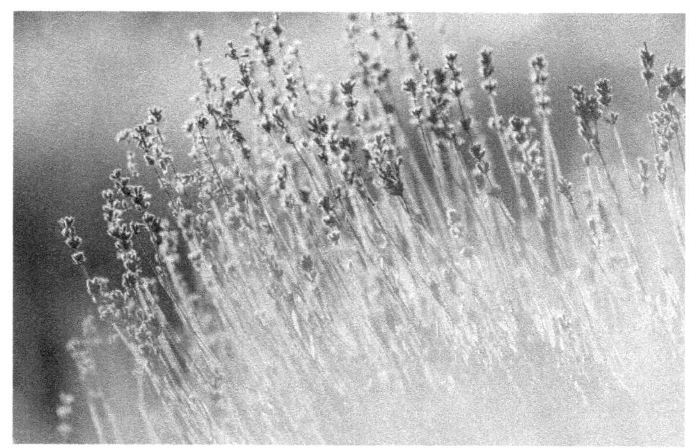

Chapter 2: Treating Acne with Herbal Remedies

Acne is a common and often distressing skin condition that can cause psychological distress or physical discomfort. The good news is that there are effective treatments for acne that can help reduce or even eliminate its appearance. Herbal remedies can provide an effective, natural and safe treatment option for people looking to clear their skin of acne. Herbal remedies for acne are derived from plants and have been used for centuries to treat skin diseases. These herbal remedies can help improve acne symptoms and are often gentler on the skin than over-the-counter medications or prescription medications. Common herbal remedies used to treat acne include green tea extract, aloe vera, tea tree oil, witch hazel, and chamomile.

When using any herbal remedy, it is important to do a patch test to make sure that your skin does not react poorly. In addition, if you are pregnant or breastfeeding, always consult your doctor before using any herbal remedy to make sure it is safe for you.

Overall, herbal remedies can be a safe and effective way to help improve the symptoms of acne. When used correctly, these remedies can help reduce the appearance of breakouts, reduce inflammation, and even help speed up healing time.

A 7-day Herbal Recipes Plan

Day 1

Recipe: Make your own acne clearing toner

Ingredients:

- 2 tablespoons of apple cider vinegar

- 2 cups of rose water

- 2 drops of tea tree oil

Instructions:

1. In a glass jar, combine the Apple Cider Vinegar and Rose Water.

2. Add the two drops of Tea tree oil and stir the mixture until the oils are blended in.

3. Store in a cool place.

Application: Apply twice a day to the affected area using a cotton pad.

Day 2

Recipe: Facial Mask for Treating Acne

Ingredients:

- 2 tablespoons of plain yoghourt

- 1 teaspoon of honey

- 1/2 teaspoon of turmeric

Instructions:

1. Mix the yoghurt, honey, and turmeric together until a thick paste has formed.

2. Apply the mixture onto your face.

3. Leave the mask on for 15-20 minutes.

4. Rinse with lukewarm water.

Application: Apply to face twice a week.

Day 3

Recipe: Acne Spot Treatment

Ingredients:

- 1 tablespoon of Aloe Vera Gel

- 1 teaspoon of raw honey

Instructions:

1. In a small bowl, mix the aloe vera and honey together until they are combined.

2. Apply the mixture directly onto your acne-prone areas.

Application: Apply twice a day to affected areas.

Day 4

Recipe: Acne-Clearing Oil Cleanser

Ingredients:

- 2 tablespoons of jojoba oil

- 2 drops of tea tree essential oil

Instructions:

1. In a small jar, combine the jojoba oil and tea tree essential oil.

2. Massage the oil cleanser onto your face for a few minutes.

3. Remove the oil with a hot, damp washcloth.

Application: Use this oil cleanser every day to help cleanse and soothe acne-prone skin.

Day 5

Recipe: Green Tea Toner

Ingredients:

- 2 green tea bags

- 2 cups of water

Instructions:

1. Place the two tea bags and the two cups of water in a small pot on high heat.

2. Once the water is boiling, turn off the heat and allow the tea to steep for 15 minutes.

3. Remove the tea bags and cool the tea down.

4. Place the tea into a glass bottle.

Application: Apply them to your face using a cotton pad, twice a day.

Day 6

Recipe: Mint Face Mask

Ingredients:

- 2 tablespoons of Greek yoghourt

- 2 tablespoons of mint leaves

Instructions:

1. In a blender, blend the Greek yoghourt and mint leaves together until a paste forms.

2. Apply the mask to your face and let sit for 15 minutes.

3. Rinse the mask off with warm water.

Application: Use this mask once a week to help reduce acne and inflammation.

Day 7

Recipe: Honey Lemon Mask

Ingredients:

- 1 tablespoons of raw honey

- 1 teaspoon of lemon juice

Instructions:

1. In a small bowl, mix the honey and lemon juice together.

2. Apply the mixture to your skin and leave it on for 15 minutes.

3. Rinse the mask off with warm water.

Application: Use this mask weekly to help with the removal of excess oils and clear up your skin.

Chapter 3: Treating Eczema with Herbal Remedies

Eczema, also known as atopic dermatitis, is a chronic inflammation of the skin that can cause itching and rash. It can occur on any part of the body, but is most commonly found on the face, hands, elbows, and knees. While there is no single cause of eczema, it is believed to be related to an overactive immune response to certain environmental triggers. Though there is currently no cure for eczema, there are many effective treatments available, including herbal remedies.

Herbal remedies have been used for centuries to treat many health conditions, including eczema. Some of the most beneficial herbs for eczema include calendula, a flowering plant known for its anti-inflammatory and anti-bacterial properties; licorice root, which is thought to prevent histamine release and reduce inflammation; and evening primrose oil, which contains omega-6 essential fatty acids that are beneficial for skin health.

A 7-day Herbal Recipes Plan

Day 1 - Chamomile Tea

Ingredients:

- 1 teaspoon of dried chamomile

- 1 cup of water

Preparation and use:

- Bring the cup of water to a boil in a small saucepan.

- Add the dried chamomile and steep for 8 – 10 minutes.

- Strain the tea and let cool to a gentle warmth.

- Dip a cotton wool ball or a clean cloth into the tea and apply it to the affected area. Leave on the skin for 15 minutes before rinsing off with lukewarm water.

Day 2 - Oatmeal Bath

Ingredients:

-1 cup of oatmeal

- Lukewarm bath water

Preparation and use:

- Grind the oatmeal into a fine powder with a coffee grinder or blender.

- Combine the oatmeal powder with lukewarm running bath water.

- Soak in the bath for up to 20 minutes.

Day 3 - Aloe Vera Gel

Ingredients:

- 1/4 cup of fresh aloe vera

Preparation and use:

- Remove the skin from the aloe vera leaf and extract the gel using a spoon

- Dab a generous amount of aloe vera gel onto the affected area and leave it on the skin to dry.

Day 4 – Licorice Root

Ingredients:

- 1 teaspoon of dried licorice root

- 1 cup of water

Preparation and use:

- Boil the water in a pan and add the dried licorice root.

- Simmer for 10-15 minutes.

- Strain the tea and let it cool before dipping a cotton cloth into it and applying it to the affected area.

- Leave it on the skin for up to 30 minutes before rinsing off with lukewarm water.

Day 5 – Cold Compress

Ingredients:

- 2 cups of cold water

- 1 clean cloth

Preparation and use:

- Bring the two cups of water to a boil in a small pan.

- Allow to cool and then add the cloth to the cold water.

- Squeeze out excess water and apply to the affected area.

- Leave on the skin for up to 15 minutes.

Day 6 – Coconut Oil

Ingredients:

- 1 teaspoon of coconut oil

Preparation and use:

- Take the teaspoon of coconut oil and apply it directly to the affected area.

- Massage the oil into the skin in a circular motion for up to 10 minutes.

Day 7 – Tea Tree Oil

Ingredients:

- 1 teaspoon of tea tree oil

- 2 tablespoons of olive oil

Preparation and use:

- Mix the tea tree oil with the olive oil and then apply a small amount to the affected area.

- Massage the oil into the skin for up to 10 minutes.

- Rinse off with lukewarm water after use.

Chapter 4: Treating Ageing Skin with Herbal Remedies

Ageing skin can be difficult to manage, as skin dullness, wrinkles, and sagging can develop with age. But there are ways to help maintain the health of ageing skin using herbal remedies. Herbal remedies are derived from plants and offer natural solutions to treating ageing skin without using harsh chemicals.

Herbal remedies contain potent antioxidants which help to improve the skin's cellular health, reduce sun damage, and even out skin tone. The antioxidants also protect the skin from free radical damage, which can cause premature ageing.

Antioxidants in herbal remedies can also help stimulate the production of collagen in the skin. Collagen is an important component of skin health as it helps to maintain skin's moisture and elasticity. Lessening the appearance of wrinkles and fine lines.

Some of the best herbal remedies for ageing skin include rosehip, calendula, neem, turmeric, and aloe vera. Rosehip oil is an excellent source of antioxidants which help to repair sun damage. Calendula has anti-inflammatory properties which help to calm irritated and red skin. Neem is a powerful antioxidant that helps reduce dark spots and protects against environmental toxins. Turmeric helps to reduce pigmentation and even out skin tone. And aloe vera helps to hydrate and soothe ageing skin.

A 7-day Herbal Recipes Plan

Day 1:

Day 1's herbal recipe is a soothing Chamomile Facial Steam:

Ingredients:

- 2 heaping teaspoons of chamomile flowers

- 2 cups of boiled water

Instructions:

- Put your chamomile flowers in a bowl, and pour the boiled water over it.

- Allow the chamomile flowers to steep in the water for about 10 minutes, stirring occasionally.

- Place your face over the bowl, making sure that your face is at least 10 inches away from the bowl, and cover your head with a towel.

- Take deep breaths and relax, allowing the steam to seep into your skin for 10-15 minutes.

- Once finished, rinse your face with cool water and pat dry.

Day 2:

Day 2's herbal recipe is a Nourishing Olive Oil & Rosemary Face Mask:

Ingredients:

- 1 tablespoon of olive oil

- 1 teaspoon of rosemary essential oil

- 2 drops of vitamin E oil

Instructions:

- In a small bowl, mix together the olive oil, rosemary essential oil, and vitamin E oil.

- Gently apply the mixture to your face and neck.

- Allow the face mask to sit for 10-15 minutes.

- Rinse the face mask off with lukewarm water and pat dry.

Day 3:

Day 3's herbal recipe is a Calming Rose & Witch Hazel Skin Toner:

Ingredients:

- 1/4 cup of rose water

- 1/4 cup of witch hazel

Instructions:

- Combine equal parts of rose water and witch hazel in a glass bottle.

- Shake it up to mix the two ingredients together.

- Soak a cotton ball in the toner and gently apply it to your face and neck.

- Allow the toner to sit for 10-15 minutes before rinsing it off with lukewarm water.

Day 4:

Day 4's herbal recipe is a Brightening Honey & Lemon Mask:

Ingredients:

- 1 tablespoon of honey

- 1 teaspoon of lemon juice

Instructions:

- In a small bowl, mix together the honey and lemon juice until it forms a paste.

- Gently apply the mixture to your face and neck.

- Allow the face mask to sit for 10-15 minutes.

- Rinse the face mask off with lukewarm water and pat dry.

Day 5:

Day 5's herbal recipe is a Hydrating Avocado Face Mask:

Ingredients:

- 1/2 an avocado

- 2 tablespoons of plain yogurt

Instructions:

- Mash the avocado and mix in the plain yoghurt.

- Gently apply the mixture to your face and neck.

- Allow the face mask to sit for 10-15 minutes.

- Rinse the face mask off with lukewarm water and pat dry.

Day 6:

Day 6's herbal recipe is a Wrinkle-Reducing Aloe Vera Mask:

Ingredients:

- 2 tablespoons of aloe vera gel

- 2 drops of lavender essential oil

Instructions:

- In a small bowl, mix together the aloe vera gel and lavender essential oil until it forms a paste.

- Gently apply the mixture to your face and neck.

- Allow the face mask to sit for 10-15 minutes.

- Rinse the face mask off with lukewarm water and pat dry.

Day 7:

Day 7's herbal recipe is a Clarifying Turmeric Mask:

Ingredients:

- 1 teaspoon of turmeric powder

- 1 tablespoon of plain yoghourt

- 2 drops of lemon essential oil

Instructions:

- In a small bowl, mix together the turmeric powder, plain yoghurt, and lemon essential oil until it forms a paste.

- Gently apply the mixture to your face and neck.

- Allow the face mask to sit for 10-15 minutes.

- Rinse the face mask off with lukewarm water and pat dry.

Chapter 5: Treating Psoriasis with herbal remedies

Psoriasis is a chronic and often debilitating skin condition that affects millions of people all around the world.

The primary symptom of psoriasis is patches of sore, inflamed skin, often in areas such as the scalp, elbows, and knees. These can be accompanied by symptoms of itching, burning, and dryness. While there is currently no known cure for psoriasis, there are several treatments which can help manage its symptoms.

One of the most popular treatments for psoriasis is herbal remedies. Herbs have been used for centuries to treat various ailments, and modern research has certainly demonstrated the medicinal properties of many herbs. Herbal remedies can be used to treat the symptoms of psoriasis, as well as fight inflammation and help to reduce the skin patches.

A 7-day Herbal Recipes Plan

Day 1

Recipe: Psoriasis Tea

Ingredients:

- 1 teaspoon of burdock root
- 1 teaspoon of Oregon grape root
- 1 teaspoon of red clover
- 1 teaspoon of cleavers
- 1 teaspoon of nettle
- 2-3 cups of boiling water

Instructions:

1. In a pot, add boiling water and all herbs.

2. Simmer for 10-15 minutes or until the water has reduced by half.

3. Strain the herbs and enjoy the tea.

Day 2

Recipe: Psoriasis Salve

Ingredients:

- 4 tablespoons of Shea Butter
- 1 tablespoon of beeswax

- 2 tablespoons of walnut oil

- 1 teaspoon of calendula oil

- 1 teaspoon of St. John's Wort oil

- 1 teaspoon of comfrey oil

- 1 teaspoon of lavender essential oil

Instructions:

1. In a double boiler, gently melt the Shea Butter and Beeswax together.

2. Remove from heat and add the walnut oil, calendula oil, St. John's Wort oil, and comfrey oil.

3. Stir until fully incorporated and then add the lavender essential oil.

4. Pour into a glass jar or container and let it cool for 1 hour before applying.

Day 3

Recipe: Psoriasis Soaking Treatment

Ingredients:

- 2-3 tablespoons of Epsom salts

- 2-3 tablespoons of sea salt

- 1 teaspoon of burdock root

- 1 teaspoon of marshmallow root

• 2-3 cups of warm water

Instructions:

1. In a bathtub or bowl, add warm water and Epsom salts, sea salt, burdock root, and marshmallow root.

2. Soak for 15-20 minutes, or until the water has cooled.

3. Pat skin dry and apply a moisturiser afterwards.

Day 4

Recipe: Psoriasis Detoxifying Bath

Ingredients:

• 2-3 tablespoons of bentonite clay

• 2-3 tablespoons of Epsom salts

• 1 tablespoon of dried calendula flowers

• 2-3 cups of warm water

Instructions:

1. In a bathtub or bowl, add warm water, bentonite clay, Epsom salts, and calendula flowers.

2. Soak for 15-20 minutes or until the water has cooled.

3. Pat skin dry and apply a moisturiser afterwards.

Day 5

Recipe: Ground Oatmeal Skin Mask

Ingredients:

• 2 tablespoon of ground oatmeal

• 1 tablespoon of honey

• 1 teaspoon of almond oil

• 1 teaspoon of aloe vera gel

Instructions:

1. In a bowl, mix all ingredients until a thick paste is formed.

2. Apply the paste to the affected area and leave on for 10-15 minutes.

3. Rinse off with warm water, pat the area dry, and apply a moisturiser afterwards.

Day 6

Recipe: Skin Soothing Herbal Infusion

Ingredients:

• 2-3 tablespoons of chamomile

• 2-3 tablespoons of lavender

• 2-3 tablespoons of calendula

• 2-3 cups of steaming hot water

Instructions:

1. In a bowl or pot, add the herbs and steaming hot water.

2. Steep for 10-15 minutes or until the water has cooled.

3. Strain the herbs and use the infusion as a skin wash or facial mist.

Day 7

Recipe: Soothing Herbal Body Oil

Ingredients:

- ½ Cup of almond oil
- 1 teaspoon of vitamin E oil
- 1 teaspoon of lavender essential oil
- 1 teaspoon of St. John's Wort oil
- 1 teaspoon of calendula oil
- 1 teaspoon of marshmallow root oil

Instructions:

1. In a bowl, mix all ingredients.

2. Transfer the oil to a container or bottle and use after showering.

3. Gently massage it onto affected areas of the skin

Chapter 6: Treating Burns and Sunburns with Herbal Remedies

Burns and sunburns are common injuries that can cause significant discomfort and damage to the skin. While conventional treatments are effective, herbal remedies offer natural alternatives that can promote healing and provide relief.

Types of Burns and Sunburns

Burns are categorised into different degrees based on their severity:

- First-degree burns affect the outer layer of the skin (epidermis), causing redness and pain.

- Second-degree burns extend into the dermis, causing blisters and more intense pain.

- Third-degree burns affect deeper tissues, potentially causing nerve damage and requiring medical attention.

Sunburns, caused by overexposure to UV radiation, typically present as a first-degree burn but can escalate with prolonged exposure.

Herbal Remedies for Burns and Sunburns

For first-degree burns and mild sunburns, aloe vera can be particularly soothing and effective. Applying fresh aloe vera gel to the affected area helps cool the skin and reduce inflammation. Lavender essential oil, when diluted in a carrier oil, can also provide relief by helping to relieve pain and prevent infection.

Calendula ointment or salve is another excellent option, aiding in reducing inflammation and speeding up the healing process. Additionally, honey is renowned for its antimicrobial properties and can be gently applied to burns to prevent infection and promote healing.

For sunburns, chamomile tea, once brewed and cooled, can be applied to the skin to soothe redness and irritation. Cucumber paste provides immediate cooling relief and reduces swelling. Similarly, green tea can be used to reduce inflammation and promote healing.

Other effective remedies include applying coconut oil, which moisturises and soothes the skin, and using witch hazel, known for its anti-inflammatory properties. You can also consider using peppermint oil, which provides a cooling sensation and helps alleviate pain. St. John's wort oil is beneficial for its healing properties, and comfrey ointment can aid in the rapid healing of damaged skin.

A 7-day Herbal Recipes Plan

Day 1 & 2: Cooling Relief Compress

- **Ingredients:**
  - 2 cups Witch Hazel (astringent, cools)
  - 1/2 cup Aloe Vera Gel (soothes, heals)
  - 5 drops Lavender Essential Oil (calming, reduces inflammation) [Note: Essential oils should be diluted before use]
- **Directions:**
  - Combine witch hazel, aloe vera gel, and lavender oil in a spray bottle.
  - Chill for 30 minutes.
  - Mist affected areas generously throughout the day.

Day 3 & 4: Soothing Oatmeal Bath

- **Ingredients:**
    - 1 cup Oatmeal (colloidal oatmeal is best, soothes)
    - 2 tablespoons Chamomile Flowers (anti-inflammatory, promotes healing)
    - 4 drops Lavender Essential Oil (optional)
- **Directions:**
    - Grind oatmeal into a fine powder (blender or food processor).
    - For ten minutes, steep chamomile flowers in boiling water.
    - Add oatmeal powder, chamomile tea, and optional lavender oil to lukewarm bathwater.
    - Soak for 20 minutes, pat dry, and avoid harsh rubbing.

Day 5 & 6: Calendula Salve

- **Ingredients:**

- 1/2 cup Infused Calendula Oil (anti-inflammatory, promotes healing) - You can purchase pre-made infused oil or make your own by steeping calendula flowers in olive oil for several weeks.
  - 1/4 cup Beeswax (forms salve base)
  - 1 tablespoon Shea Butter (moisturises)
  - 5 drops Lavender Essential Oil (optional)

- **Directions:**
  - In a double boiler, melt shea butter and beeswax.
  - Slowly whisk in calendula oil.
  - Remove from heat and let cool slightly.
  - Stir in lavender oil (optional).
  - Pour into a clean container and let it solidify.
  - A thin layer should be applied to the affected area at least 3 times a day.

Day 7: Rehydrating Mask

- **Ingredients:**
    - 1/2 ripe Avocado (moisturises, promotes healing)
    - 1 tablespoon Honey (antibacterial, soothes)
    - 1 tablespoon Plain Yogurt (soothes, provides moisture)
- **Directions:**
    - Mash avocado until smooth.
    - Stir in honey and yoghurt.
    - Apply a thick layer to the affected area and leave on for 15-20 minutes.
    - Rinse with cool water and pat dry.

Additional Tips:

- Drink plenty of fluids to stay hydrated.
- Wear loose-fitting clothing made from natural fibres.

- Avoid sun exposure until sunburn heals completely.
- Apply a gentle, fragrance-free moisturiser daily.

Remember, this is just a sample plan. You can adjust the herbs based on their availability and your preferences.

Chapter 7: Treating Hyperpigmentation with herbal remedies

Hyperpigmentation occurs when melanin, your skin's pigment, is produced in excess, creating darker patches. Sun damage, inflammation, and hormonal changes can all contribute to it.

Herbal Remedies

- **Licorice Root:** Licorice extract may help lighten skin by inhibiting tyrosinase, an enzyme involved in melanin production.
- **Green Tea:** Green tea contains antioxidants that may help reduce hyperpigmentation and protect from sun damage. You can use brewed green tea compresses or look for creams containing green tea extract.
- **Turmeric:** Curcumin, the active compound in turmeric, has anti-inflammatory and skin-lightening properties. Topical application of turmeric paste or creams

might be beneficial. Be aware turmeric can stain skin yellow.

- **Licorice Root and Mulberry:** Some studies suggest a combination of licorice and mulberry extracts may be effective for hyperpigmentation.

- Apple Cider Vinegar: Apple cider vinegar contains acetic acid, which may act as a mild exfoliant and potentially lighten skin tone. However, due to its acidity, it can irritate the skin. It's crucial to dilute it significantly (1 part vinegar to 3-4 parts water) and do a patch test before applying it to a larger area.

A 7-day Herbal Recipes Plan

Instructions:

* Always do a patch test on a small area of your inner arm before applying to a larger ar,c ea.

* Discontinue use if any irritation occurs.

* These recipes are for external use only. Do not ingest.

Day 1 & 2: Exfoliating Mask with Licorice Root In

* Ingredients:

* 1 tablespoon Licorice Root Powder (brightening)

* 1 tablespoon Gram Flour (exfoliates) [You can substitute with oatmeal]

* 1 tablespoon Plain Yogurt (soothes, provides moisture)

* 1 teaspoon Honey (antibacterial, soothes)

* **Directions**:

* Put together all ingredients in a bowl to form a paste.

* A thin layer should be applied to cleansed skin, avoiding the eye area.

* Leave on for 15 minutes.

* Rinse off with cool water and pat dry.

* Follow with a gentle moisturiser.

Day 3 & 4: Green Tea Toner

* Ingredients:

* 2 Green Tea Bags (antioxidant, reduces hyperpigmentation)

* 1 cup Hot Water

* 1 tablespoon Apple Cider Vinegar (diluted - 1 part vinegar to 3 parts water) (brightening, exfoliates - use with caution)

* Directions:

* Put green tea bags in hot water for about 10 minutes.

* Tea bags should be removed and let cool completely.

* Stir in diluted apple cider vinegar.

* Toner should be applied to the cleansed skin with a cotton pad.

* Allow to air dry or rinse with cool water and pat dry.

* Follow with a moisturiser.

Day 5 & 6: Turmeric Paste

* Ingredients:

* 1 tablespoon Turmeric Powder (brightening, anti-inflammatory)

* 1 tablespoon Plain Yogurt (soothes, provides moisture)

* 1 teaspoon Honey (antibacterial, soothes)

* Directions:

* Put together all ingredients in a bowl to form a paste.

* Apply a thin layer to cleansed skin, avoiding the eye area (turmeric can stain).

* Leave on for 15 minutes.

* Rinse off with cool water and pat dry.

* Follow with a moisturiser.

Day 7: Hydrating Mask with Mulberry

* Ingredients:

    * 1 tablespoon Mulberry Powder (brightening)

    * 1/2 ripe Avocado (moisturises)

    * 1 tablespoon Honey (antibacterial, soothes)

* Directions:

    * Mash avocado until smooth.

* Stir in mulberry powder and honey.

* A thick layer should be applied to cleansed skin and should be left on for 15-20 minutes.

* Rinse off with cool water and pat dry.

Additional Tips:

* Wash skin with a gentle cleanser morning and night.

* Apply a broad-spectrum sunscreen (SPF 30 or higher) daily, even on cloudy days.

* Avoid sun exposure during peak hours (10 am to 4 pm).

* Consider incorporating antioxidant-rich foods like fruits and vegetables into your diet.

Conclusion

Herbal remedies have many potential benefits for treating skin conditions. They are typically natural, low-cost, accessible, and cause fewer side-effects and adverse reactions than some modern pharmaceutical treatments. Plant-based compounds like various fruits, herbs, and oils have been used to treat skin conditions since ancient times. In modern times, research has shown that some herbal remedies can be effective in treating conditions like acne, eczema, psoriasis, and wrinkles. Herbal remedies can be taken orally or used externally as lotions, masks, and creams, and often provide relief without causing irritation to the skin. Furthermore, these remedies provide a more holistic approach to skin care, aiming to improve skin health from the inside out. Although further research is needed to better understand the effectiveness of herbal treatments for skin conditions, the evidence to date suggests that they may be a safe and, potentially, effective way to help manage various skin problems.

www.ingramcontent.com/pod-product-compliance
Lightning Source LLC
Chambersburg PA
CBHW072342270726
48659CB00023B/2207